Eating Right for Life
Prostate Cancer Nutrition & You

3

D1611700

Editorial Director: Elsie Wagner
Editor: Jackie Rosenhek
Production Manager: Danielle Leblanc
Art Direction and Design: Julie Margot, Pierre Marc Pelletier
President & Publisher: Madeleine Partous

©2000
Eating Right for Life is published
by Parkhurst, 400 McGill Street,
3rd Floor, Montréal, Québec, H2Y 2G1.

Publication of this book is made
possible by an unrestricted
educational grant from
Abbott Laboratories, Limited.

Prostate cancer and the diet factor

If you were one of the 19,000 Canadian men diagnosed with prostate cancer this year, then you've already faced some difficult treatment decisions. You may also be wondering if there's anything else you can do — any other choices you can make to decrease your risk of recurrence, no matter what therapy you're undergoing. The good news is that all signs point towards *yes*.

As with other cancers, a few important "risk factors" are linked to prostate cancer — age, hormones, race and genes all play a role. For example, the disease seems to progress more rapidly in some groups, such as people of African descent, than in others. Likewise, your risk of developing prostate cancer is two to five times higher if your brother or father is affected. Unfortunately, these are the types of things we're born with; after all, you can't very well change your family history at this point! But there is at least one risk factor you *can* do something about — your diet.

Cause and effect

Current research in prostate cancer suggests that changes in so-called modifiable risk factors, such as diet, may translate into very meaningful benefits. Like all cancers, prostate cancer is caused by genetic mutation. Genetic mutations are either inherited or acquired through exposure to harmful substances in our environment (for example, we know that cigarette smoke can lead to lung cancer). Although inherited factors are important in some prostate cancers, the overwhelming majority are related to the environment — and diet seems to be key. A host of observations forms the basis of this belief, especially when researchers look at the international variance in prostate cancer incidence.

Prostate cancer is the most commonly diagnosed cancer among men living in the Westernized World, such as Canada, the United States, Northern Europe and Australia. In other nations, however, prostate cancer is rarely diagnosed. This mostly includes countries in the Pacific Rim (such as Japan, China, Taiwan and

Thailand), several Middle Eastern countries and Northern Africa. A Japanese man, for example, is 10 times less likely to die from prostate cancer than a typical North American man. Men from Thailand are a whopping 100 times less likely! By looking at the world-wide differences in cancer rates, we see that prostate cancer is either related to environmental factors, such as diet, or due to the unique genetic make-up of a country's citizens.

Nature or nurture?

But which is it — genes or environment? "Migration" studies may offer some answers. After examining the prostate cancer rates among people who move from low-risk countries like China and Japan to high-risk areas like Canada, researchers discovered that their risk of prostate cancer rises. Not only that, but the children of these immigrants have almost the same chance of developing prostate cancer as the locals. These studies suggest that it's the environment or lifestyle elements, such as diet, as opposed to inherited traits, that are largely responsible for the disease. If genetics were a more important factor, then Chinese and Japanese Canadians would be at low risk for prostate cancer — but they're not.

Although we don't yet know the full relationship between the food we eat and prostate cancer, the news is encouraging. This book is designed to guide you through the process of changing your eating habits for the better, in the hopes of helping fight the cancer and improving your overall health. Who knows? You might even like it!

5

Important note:

This book is our best attempt to offer nutritional counselling related to prostate cancer. But because the research is yet incomplete, you should know that we cannot make any claims that following this diet plan will, in fact, help or harm you. **Men currently taking medications and/or men with pre-existing health conditions, such as kidney disease or diabetes, should consult their physicians before undertaking a diet change or taking nutritional supplements.** The suggestions in this book are not meant in any way to replace treatment or therapy suggested by your doctor, but rather to complement them.

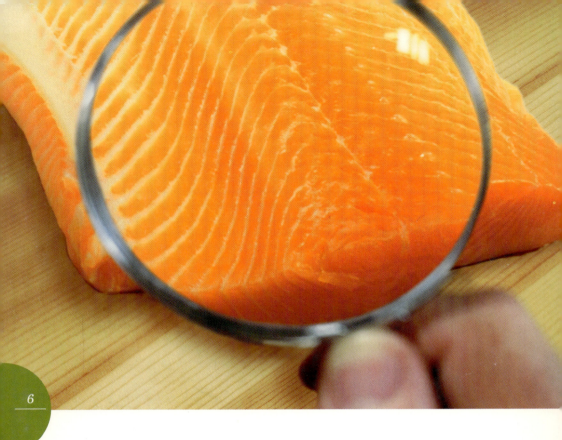

Fat and protein:
Looking for the right balance

1 **Fat and protein are essential parts of any balanced diet — but they're also key elements in the development of prostate cancer.**

Although your body needs some fat to function properly and absorb nutrients from the foods you eat, there's a strong link between dietary fat intake and the risk of developing prostate cancer. There's convincing evidence that men with prostate cancer who eat higher amounts of fat experience more rapid cancer growth.

Getting enough protein is also crucial, and that can be diffi-

cult — especially if you're cutting down on meat and dairy products, the traditional sources of protein in Western diets. These
so-called animal proteins, while high in protein, are
also high in fat. The solution? Plant protein — a
low-fat and versatile source of the protein your
body needs. Of all the plant proteins available, soy
is the most complete, offering a full range of essential amino acids and "cancer-fighting" isoflavones.

In China and Japan, the traditional diet has 15 to 20 percent of calories from fat. In North America, it includes 38 to 40 percent of calories from fat.

The fat factor

A low-fat diet is the first step on the road to
prostate health. In China and Japan, the traditional
diet has 15 to 20 percent of calories from fat. In North America,
the typical diet includes 38 to 40 percent of calories from fat.
Interested in this possible link between diet and prostate cancer,
researchers have been putting the theory to the test — and the
results are very convincing.

Recent studies have shown that fat or fatty foods are associated with the development of prostate cancer. When researchers
put human prostate cancer cells into mice, the cancer grows
faster if the mice eat a high-fat diet. It looks like the same might
hold true for humans: At least one study suggests that prostate
cancer is more likely to progress in men whose diet has a high fat
content. And at New York's Sloan-Kettering Cancer Center, even
men without established prostate cancer managed to reduce their
prostate-specific antigen (PSA) values by eating a low-fat diet.

Hormones and fat

Dietary fats and cholesterol are part of the
building blocks of androgens — male hormones associated with prostate-cancer
development. It's theoretically possible that
chronically elevated levels of testosterone,
the major male androgen, can lead to
prostate cancer. There's increasing evidence
that high-fat diets can increase levels of

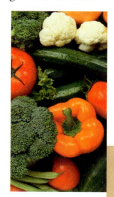

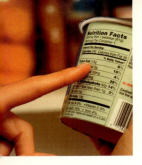

androgens. For example, vegetarians (who tend to consume less dietary fat) often have lower levels of testosterone than meat-eaters.

Steps to a low-fat diet

Get in the habit of reading food labels and choosing lower-fat options when you shop.

Eating a low-fat diet isn't hard to do. Start by avoiding fried foods, eating smaller (palm-sized) portions of meat (especially red meat), and cutting down on butter, margarine, oils and cream. Opt for more fruits and vegetables, beans and pasta, whole-grain breads, leaner cuts of meat and low-fat dairy products. Just be aware of what you're eating — and get in the habit of reading food labels and choosing lower-fat options when you shop for groceries. Pretty soon, making healthier choices will become a habit.

Protein: animal vs plant

Our bodies need protein to build tissue for growth and repair. The two sources of protein in our diets are either animal- or plant-based. We traditionally associate eating meats, fish and dairy products with good sources of protein. But the problem with these foods is that protein isn't always the main ingredient — fat is.

While meat is protein-rich, most cuts of meat are also high in fat: A T-bone steak, for example, provides only 20 percent of its calories from protein — fully 80 percent is from fat. Fish is a better source of protein because most types are naturally low in fat. Be careful, though: Canned tuna packed in oil has a 64-percent fat content, and frying any type of fish will ruin even the best of intentions (steaming, broiling or barbecuing are better options). Milk and dairy proteins, the final animal protein source, can also be very high in fat, most of it saturated (the "bad" kind).

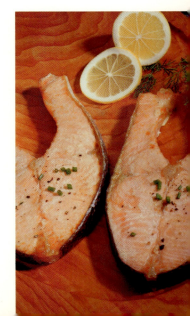

Plant power

The solution to finding the right fat-protein balance is plant protein. If we could design a perfect food, this would be it — full of vitamins and minerals, low in fat and sodium, and high in protein, carbohydrates and fibre. Best of all, plant proteins taste good and they're inexpensive. And unlike meat, they deliver carbohydrates instead of fat along with the protein. The richest sources of these amazing vegetable proteins are legumes — dried split peas and beans.

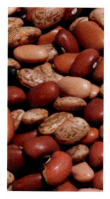

There are literally hundreds of varieties of beans. Depending on the kind, one cup of beans has 150 to 300 calories and a healthy 12 to 25 grams of protein. Kidney beans, for example, provide 25 percent of their calories from protein and 70 percent from carbohydrates. But by far the best source is the soybean, commonly consumed in the form of tofu. It's the only plant protein that contains sufficient amounts of all nine essential amino acids.

■ The soy story

There are at least two good reasons to add soy to your diet: It's a great source of low-fat protein and it also contains special ingredients called isoflavones, including genistein and daidzein — compounds likely to play an important role in holding off the growth of prostate tumours.

There are at least two good reasons to add soy to your diet: It's a great source of low-fat protein and it also contains special ingredients called isoflavones.

Studies based on the Asian population's lower prostate cancer rate show that Asians typically consume a low-fat diet filled with lots of tofu, tempeh and soy milk — all excellent sources of soy protein. Blood and urine analyses of Asian men have revealed that the samples contain anywhere from seven to 100 times more isoflavones than the samples of North American men. Plus, lab tests on

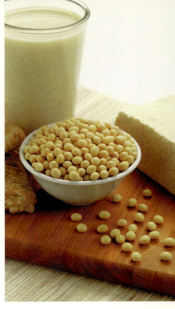

genistein, the type of isoflavone found abundantly in soy foods, show that it's a potent inhibitor of cancer cells, including prostate cancer.

■ Adding soy to your diet

After lowering your fat intake, the second most important step in a prostate-friendly diet is adding soy. Nutritionists recommend 40 grams daily, a figure established from laboratory research: Tumours grew more slowly when nutrition included 40 grams of soy protein. Yet the typical Canadian diet contains virtually no soy products. To learn more about the different types, see the box on the facing page.

Before you buy...

☛ Keep in mind that adding soy to your diet may cause you to gain a few pounds if you don't adjust your regular eating habits, although lowering your overall fat intake may help counteract any weight gain.

☛ Men who are on protein-restricted diets for medical reasons (diabetes, liver or kidney disease) should consult their doctors before adding soy to their diet.

☛ Levels of isoflavones, number of protein grams, and fat and calcium content vary widely across different brands. Read the labels carefully to select the soy products best for you.

A GLOSSARY OF SOY PRODUCTS

Tofu — a semi-soft food made from adding mineral salt to soy milk — is a handy and nutritious substitute for meat. Like all soy products, it's an excellent source of protein and is low in fat. Surely the most versatile form of soy, tofu has varying degrees of firmness (the firmer it is, the higher the fat content). The softer form is best for sauces and dips; the denser type for grilling, baking and stir-frying. Tofu lends itself well to a variety of recipes because it absorbs any flavours that are mixed in with it.

Soy milk is made from ground and cooked soybeans. The soy "milk" is filtered out during this process. It can be used as a dairy substitute — drink it straight from the carton, put it on your breakfast cereal, or use it as a replacement for milk in cooking or baking. It also comes in flavours like vanilla, strawberry and chocolate. Note: Avoid non-fat soy milk, since soybeans lose some of their beneficial properties when completely defatted. Opt for regular or low-fat varieties.

Tempeh, a textured vegetable protein (TVP) made from cooked and fermented soybeans, can also be used as a meat substitute. It's high in calcium, iron, zinc, fibre and it's cholesterol-free. Another TVP, **miso**, made from fermented soybean paste, is commonly used in soups.

Soy powder is available as flour (whole ground soy flour is best), granules or isolate. It's easy to use in cooking (just add water) and it also comes in different flavours: Mix it with fruit juices, soy milk or skim milk as a refreshing drink.

Soy sauce and **Tamari**: Most types of so-called "soy sauce" aren't made from soybeans at all — they're just coloured and flavoured water. To get the real benefit of soy, use tamari instead, which is a fermented brew made from soybeans.

11

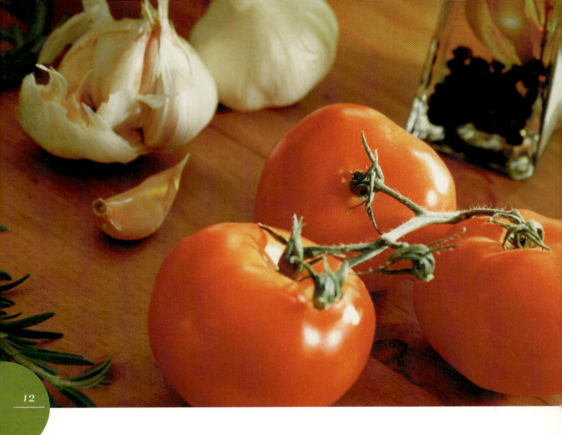

Antioxidants:
Foods that fight for you

2 **Plant-based foods have many advantages over meat. They're packed with vitamins, minerals and phytonutrients ("phyto" means plant), health-promoting compounds that interact to help your body stay healthy and fight disease.**

Most vital are those that act as antioxidants, which neutralize the DNA-damaging free-radical oxygen molecules that can lead to cancer. Vitamin E, selenium (a mineral) and a host of phytonutrients are all powerful antioxidants.

Keep in mind, though, that it takes more than just eating one

or two of these nutrients once in a while. You need to eat a varied diet **daily** that includes as many of these health-promoting
nutrients as possible. In some cases, adapting your
diet to include the right foods is all you need to do;
in others, supplementation may be the best way to
get these vitamins and minerals. In these cases, we
provide recommendations for how much of a supplement you should take.

*You need to eat a varied diet **daily** that includes as many health-promoting nutrients as possible.*

Choosing supplements

When you're in the drug or health-food store, ask about which
supplement brands come highly recommended, and read the
labels carefully yourself. Potency levels are given in International
Units (IU), milligrams (mg) or micrograms (µg), a number
clearly listed on each bottle. Also, check with your doctor about
whether the government's Recommended Daily Allowance, or
RDA, of any supplement is right for you.

Adding it up: Mixing multivitamins and supplements

If you already take a multivitamin, remember to deduct the
amount of any given nutrient from the total daily recommendation when buying additional single-nutrient supplements. For
example, if your multivitamin already contains 50 µg of selenium and you want to take 200 µg in total, take your multivitamin
and a 100-µg or a 150-µg selenium supplement, rather than a
200-µg version.

Vital vitamins

We all need vitamins for proper metabolic func-
tioning. While the amounts we need are very small,
our bodies can't manufacture most of them — they
must come from the foods we eat.

Vitamin E

Vitamin E is one of the most promising antioxidants in slowing the
progression of prostate cancer. It occurs naturally in plant-based

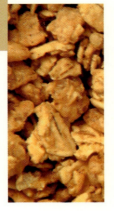

fatty foods like nuts and sunflower seeds; hazelnut, safflower, canola, corn and olive oils; wheat germ; leafy green vegetables and asparagus; mangoes; wheat germ and whole grains.

Studies have already shown that men who consume more dietary sources of Vitamin E have a lower risk of certain cancers, including prostate cancer. An added benefit: In a study of mice injected with human prostate cancer cells, vitamin E counteracted the effects of a high-fat diet — a positive result, of course, but don't think of vitamin E as the cure for an addiction to French fries!

■ **Vitamin E supplement recommendation: 400-800 IU a day**
Unfortunately, some of the best sources of Vitamin E, like nuts and oils, are very high in fat, making it difficult or unhealthy to get the full daily dose of 400 to 800 IU from foods. *Caution: Men who are taking drugs to prevent blood clotting (including aspirin) should consult their doctors first, since vitamin E also has a blood-thinning effect. For the same reason, men should not take vitamin E supplements one week before or immediately after surgery.*

Vitamin D
This isn't an ordinary vitamin — your body also turns it into an important hormone. The main function of vitamin D is to increase your body's natural production of calcium. If you get a lot of calcium from your diet, though, your body will stop producing vitamin D — and researchers have found that men with the highest calcium intake also have the highest levels of prostate cancer. Vitamin D also controls cell growth and death. In mice, scientists have been able to kill or slow the growth of prostate cancer cells by giving them vitamin D.

In mice, scientists have been able to kill or slow the growth of prostate cancer cells by giving them vitamin D.

Sunlight triggers our bodies to produce vitamin D. Men who live in northern countries — and who are exposed to less sunlight — have higher rates of prostate cancer than their

14

counterparts in the South. The primary dietary source of the vitamin is fatty fish, and it's speculated that Asians may be protected from prostate cancer because they get lots of vitamin D in their fish-heavy diets. In addition, as men age, their bodies are less able to manufacture the vitamin, perhaps leading to an increased risk of prostate cancer.

■ **Vitamin D supplement recommendation: 400 IU a day**

Consider taking this supplement only if you don't eat fish (the main source of dietary Vitamin D) or if you're not getting enough sunlight. Fifteen minutes' exposure without sunscreen — in the early morning or late afternoon — every day or so is all it takes. Don't worry: This amount of exposure isn't damaging, unless you've had skin cancer, in which case a supplement is a better idea.

Sunlight triggers the body to produce vitamin D. Fifteen minutes' exposure every day or so is all it takes.

Minerals that matter

It's now clear that minerals, like vitamins, are essential to a host of vital body processes — including the fight against cancer. Of the more than 60 minerals in the body, 22 are essential, which means that our bodies can't manufacture them. We need to get them from foods or supplements.

Selenium

This one's a crucial antioxidant. Scientists were first tipped off about its potential "cancer-fighting" benefits when they noticed that countries whose soils have low levels of selenium (like Canada) also have higher rates of cancer, including prostate cancer. A study done in the southern United States 12 years ago strongly supports the selenium-prostate cancer link. In a random group of men with skin cancer, half were given selenium and half were given a placebo. Although scientists found that the mineral didn't decrease skin cancer recurrence, they discovered a 70-percent reduction in prostate cancer in the men taking selenium! Since then, other researchers are finding similar results.

Countries whose soils have low levels of selenium (like Canada) also have higher rates of cancer, including prostate cancer.

■ **Recommended selenium supplement: 200 µg a day**

Although a healthy diet provides most people with almost all of the necessary minerals, men with prostate cancer should take selenium in "antioxidant doses" — a level virtually impossible to obtain from diet alone. (The current Recommended Daily Allowance (RDA) for men is only 70 µg). *Caution: Doses higher than 200 µg of selenium a day may be toxic and cause extra health problems, so don't exceed this limit.*

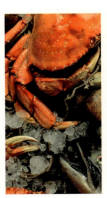

Zinc

This mineral helps our bodies repair wounds, synthesize protein, cause cells to reproduce and protect against free radicals — all to the good. But its exact function within the prostate is unknown. The mineral is found mostly in meat, poultry, eggs, liver and seafood (particularly oysters and crab meat), as well as in black-eyed peas, tofu and wheat germ. Although zinc has been touted as an important substance for the treatment of prostate disorders, there's no sound scientific evidence to back this up.

■ **Zinc supplements**

There's no need to go beyond the RDA of 15 mg, the maximum amount a multivitamin should contain if you're taking one. Natural sources of zinc — meat, poultry, seafood, tofu and wheat germ — can easily provide you with enough of the mineral. Therefore, a zinc supplement isn't recommended. If you do want to take one, don't exceed 15 mg a day.

Feisty phytonutrients

Phytonutrients aren't vitamins or minerals, but they have important health benefits. We've identified more than 4000 kinds of phytonutrients, derived only from plant sources, and more are being discovered all the time. Soy protein, for example, is one of the most important kinds. Many phytonutrients pos-

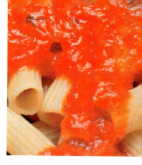

sess properties that make them very attractive in terms of preventing or limiting diseases like prostate cancer.

While vitamin and mineral supplementation makes sense in some cases, phytonutrient supplements don't exist for the most part, so it's important to eat plenty of foods from the following categories of phytonutrients.

The lycopenes in processed or cooked tomatoes are more easily absorbed by your body than the ones in fresh tomatoes.

Lycopenes

Lycopenes are a kind of antioxidant found particularly in tomatoes (it's what makes them red), as well as in papaya and watermelon. Researchers have found that men with prostate cancer have low levels of lycopenes in their blood and prostate tissue. The evidence supporting a lycopene-rich diet is very convincing — many studies suggest that men who eat more than 10 servings a week of cooked tomatoes have a one-third reduction in prostate cancer incidence.

Unlike with many other fruits and veggies, fresh isn't necessarily the way to go here: Processed tomatoes (in sauces and juices) are better than fresh ones because lycopenes are fat-soluble, which means your body will absorb more of them when processed with a little bit of oil. And cooking tomatoes is also preferred, since heat releases the lycopenes from inside the cells.

■ **Recommended lycopene supplement: 30-60 mg a day**

Lycopene is now available as a supplement. If you prefer to go the natural route, a large can of tomato juice contains 28 mg of lycopenes (opt for a low-sodium version, if possible).

Sulphoraphanes: Veggies

Cruciferous vegetables — like cabbage, broccoli, broccoli sprouts, cauliflower and brussels sprouts — are rich in sulphoraphanes, a group of antioxidant compounds that helps detoxify ingested cancer-causing compounds and flush them out of your body. The best source of naturally occurring sulphoraphane is broccoli sprouts: In fact, you'd have to eat about two pounds of broccoli to get the same amount of sulphoraphane in just a small amount of broccoli sprouts.

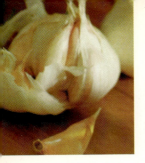

Researchers found that letting fresh garlic stand for 15 minutes before cooking it activates its cancer-fighting enzymes.

18

Alliums: Garlic and more

Garlic has received much attention in the press with respect to its "anti-cancer" properties. Indeed, the scientific evidence points towards increasing your garlic intake: People who ate garlic-containing foods two or more times a week had about half the risk of developing prostate cancer. Garlic belongs to a family of vegetables known as alliums, which also includes leeks, shallots and chives. These vegetables can help fight prostate cancer in a variety of ways. Aside from their antioxidant properties, they can enhance the disposal of cancer-causing chemicals and protect DNA from harmful substances. Allium vegetables are also a good source of selenium.

Opt for foods made with fresh garlic instead of taking supplements, since lots of synthesized compounds are added by manufacturers whenever garlic is chopped, crushed or minced. After crushing fresh garlic, let it stand for 15 minutes before cooking with it — researchers have found that this activates a "cancer-fighting" enzyme within. On the other hand, roasting garlic in the peel may taste great, but heating it in this way destroys the enzyme.

Omega-3 fatty acids

These nutrients play an important role in maintaining a healthy prostate and repairing diseased tissue. They're found mostly in fatty fish like salmon, trout, anchovies, sardines, bluefish and white albacore tuna. Other sources of omega-3 fatty acids are leafy green vegetables, tofu, walnuts, canola oil and flaxseed oil (the richest plant source). We know that omega-3 fatty acids can inhibit the growth of human prostate cancer cells in a test tube. Eating fish twice a week, the evidence suggests, may be enough to reap these positive benefits.

■ **Omega-3 fatty acid supplements:**
Natural sources like fish are the best way to get enough omega-3 fatty acids. If you do want to take a supplement, though, don't exceed 200 to 400 IU a day. *Caution: Men with*

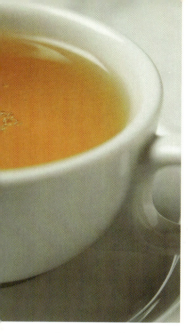

a family history of stroke, diabetes or who are on blood-thinning medications (including aspirin) could, in rare instances, experience side effects from supplementing with these oils, and should consult their doctors first.

Polyphenols: Green tea and soy

These powerful antioxidants may inhibit tumour growth. One of the best ways to add polyphenols to your diet is to drink green tea, a favourite in many Asian countries where men have low rates of prostate cancer. Studies show that drinking three to 10 cups of green tea a day coincides with reduced levels of certain cancers, and polyphenols may also help prevent the cellular damage that can lead to prostate cancer. It's no wonder: The polyphenols found in green tea can be up to several hundred times more powerful than those found in Vitamin E.

Among the richest food sources of these beneficial polyphenols are the skins of purple or red grapes or berries — so go ahead and have a glass of red wine (or grape juice, for the less adventurous). And finally, some good news for chocoholics: Studies have found significant levels of polyphenols in chocolate and cocoa products. But read the labels: It's important to choose products with a high content of real cocoa butter or powder — and don't overdo it, since chocolate is mostly fat.

And remember isoflavones, those "anti-cancer" compounds found in soy? Well, they're also a type of polyphenol with powerful antioxidant properties.

■ Recommended soy supplement: 40 grams a day

As mentioned in Chapter 1, if you're finding it hard to include soy in your diet, soy-protein supplements are available in the form of powders and tasty pre-mixed drinks.

19

The skins of purple or red grapes are rich sources of beneficial polyphenols — so go ahead and have a glass of red wine.

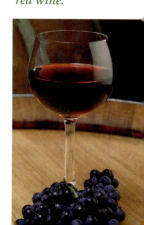

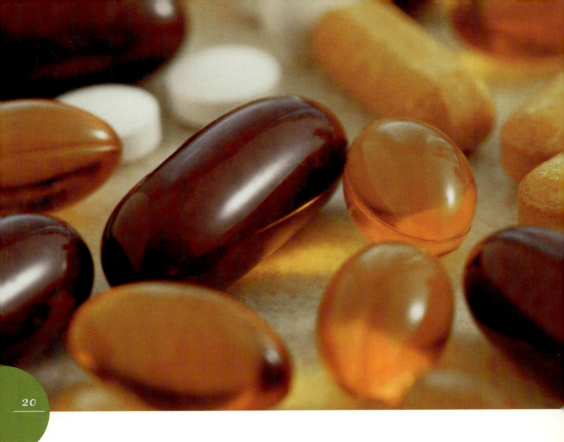

Supplements:
The good, the bad and the iffy

3

Now that you're familiar with the most crucial vitamins, minerals and phytonutrients, the question becomes: How do you get the right amount of each?

In an ideal world, simply eating a well-balanced diet would be enough. But sometimes that's just not possible. Supplements — manufactured, easy-to-take versions of these nutrients — may be the answer. Although there's no firm data that dietary supplements can cure or prevent prostate cancer, evidence suggests that some may help slow tumour growth — the ultimate goal in managing the disease. But take note: Too much of certain vitamins can actually be

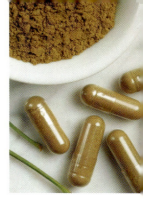

harmful to the prostate. And there are also countless less familiar supplements out there, including herbal preparations, that make a variety of claims — some true, others not. Below you'll find details on which supplements we recommend and which ones we don't, as well as the low-down on the most popular herbal products.

Herbal products and other supplements

Lots of big claims are made by manufacturers of herbal products, and those geared towards men with prostate cancer are no exception. Literally dozens of "alternative" — often untested — remedies for prostate cancer are already selling like hotcakes on the Internet. If you do decide to take a herbal or alternative supplement, don't rely on "testimonials": Remember that the supplement industry isn't regulated, and keep in mind that many of these products may actually do more harm than good. And before you take any new supplement, herbal or otherwise, consult your doctor. Here's the story on some of the most popular — and hyped — alternative products.

Before you take any new supplement, herbal or otherwise, consult your doctor.

Melatonin

This hormone regulates the body's sleep-wake cycle, but some recent evidence suggests that it also possesses some anti-cancer properties, including those potentially beneficial in fighting prostate cancer. In one study, which compared melatonin levels in men with and without prostate cancer, the men with prostate cancer showed evidence of a melatonin deficiency. But will taking a supplement offer any benefits? We simply don't know for sure, although the results seem promising. In another study, men with hormone-refractory prostate cancer that couldn't be treated conventionally were controlled with high-dose melatonin. Other studies are currently underway.

Melatonin does have the potential to do harm, however. The non-synthetic variety of the supplement is derived from cows' brains, and carries a theoretical risk of transmitting illnesses like mad-cow disease. So, should you take melatonin supplements? Until the results of more conclusive studies come in, the answer is probably no.

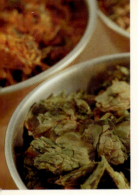

Some herbal treatments may do more harm than good.

Prostate cancer-SPES

This combination of eight herbs — chrysanthemum, licorice, isatis, Ganoderma lucidum, Panax pseudo-ginseng, Rabdosia rubescens, saw palmetto and scutellaria (skullcap) — is gaining popularity among prostate-cancer patients. In a paper published in the *New England Journal of Medicine*, eight patients with hormone-sensitive prostate cancer were given PC-SPES. In all patients, testosterone and PSA levels fell. This suggests that PC-SPES may have hormone-like properties and may even have some anti-prostate cancer properties.

Although this may sound good, all patients developed the typical signs of "estrogenization": They became impotent and their breasts became tender. One patient even developed a blood clot in the leg — a well-known and potentially fatal complication of high-dose estrogen treatment. When considering this therapy for hormone-sensitive cancers, opt for traditional pharmacological forms of androgen deprivation instead (like LHRH hormonal therapy), especially since there are fewer side effects — and it makes no sense to use an unproven concoction.

Shark cartilage

While no evidence exists that supplements of shark cartilage have any beneficial effect on prostate cancer, there are some findings that suggest it may reduce the development of blood vessels that feed tumours and tumour metastasis. Until the results are in, steer clear.

Saw palmetto: Help or hype?

Saw palmetto is the partially dried, ripe fruit of a scrubby palm that grows in the South-Eastern United States. More false information has been published on this plant than on just about any other prostate cancer remedy. Although there's evidence that saw palmetto is beneficial for symptoms of prostatism, studies that support its actual anti-cancer claims are often flawed and yield inconsistent results, and the long-term results of taking the substance aren't yet known. More respectable studies have found only inconclusive results as to its benefits. In addition, the product quality varies alarmingly from one manufacturer to another. Our investigation of available saw palmetto supplements revealed, according to product labels, a tenfold difference in active ingredients (known as liposterolic extracts, or fatty acids and sterols) across brands. (Theoretically, the supplements are supposed to contain 85 to 95 percent of these extracts to be effective.)

Studies that support saw palmetto's anti-cancer claims are often flawed and yield inconsistent results.

Supplements to avoid
Vitamin A as beta-carotene

Since more than one study has found a higher risk of various types of cancer associated with high-dose beta-carotene supplements, they should be avoided. But that said, it doesn't mean you should avoid naturally occurring beta-carotene from food sources — yellow, orange, red and dark green fruits and vegetables like cantaloupe, carrots, spinach, sweet potatoes and broccoli. These foods are good for you, and the beta-carotene they contain is safe and beneficial. And since one medium carrot a day contains all the beta-carotene you need (no more than the Recommended Daily Allowance (RDA) of 5000 IU), there's really no need for a supplement.

Calcium

Adequate calcium is essential to build and maintain strong bones, but recent findings have revealed an association between excessive calcium intake and a possible tripling of the risk of prostate cancer. So it makes sense for men with prostate cancer to avoid supplements, and to get the RDA of calcium from their diets instead — 800 mg per day for men who don't have osteoporosis. *Caution: Some soy drinks and shakes are fortified with calcium, so opt for unfortified versions instead.*

DHEA or dihydrepiandrostenedione

This sounds scary, and for good reason — men with prostate cancer should definitely avoid this one. DHEA, which has received lots of press in relation to weightlifting, is a steroidal androgen produced by the adrenal gland. As an androgen, it helps stimulate muscle generation, but may also stimulate the growth of prostate cancer cells.

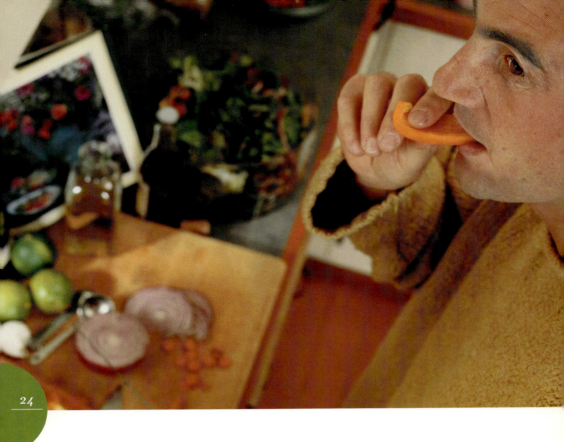

Hormonal and radiation therapies: Nutrition and your treatment program

4

Depending on the type of treatment you're receiving, you may need to consider special nutritional factors.

Also, any drugs you may be taking in conjunction with your treatment program can have side effects of their own — like altering your mood or taste — which in turn may reduce your interest in eating properly. The best way to stay on top of all these things is to consult your doctor about nutrition and how it relates to you.

Radiation therapy

Lots of men receive radiation therapy as part of their prostate cancer treatment plan. It can be given via external x-ray beams (known as external beam radiotherapy) or using internally placed radiation sources such as radioactive iodine or palladium (known as brachytherapy).

It seems like a good idea to limit your consumption of antioxidants during radiation therapy.

Radiation treatment is based on the concept of using "oxidative kill" to destroy prostate cancer cells. The radiation, once in contact with the cells, generates toxic oxygen — free radicals which then cause permanent damage to the cells' DNA. If this process sounds familiar, it's because prostate cancer itself may be caused by a similar mechanism. But how can the very thing that's part of what causes cancer be used to treat it? The answer is that it may simply be an issue of the "dose" of oxygen damage. Small amounts will damage DNA and cause non-lethal cell injury — possibly resulting in cancer formation — whereas large doses kill the cells entirely.

With radiation therapy, the implications on nutrition are potentially profound. Since most of the foods and nutritional supplements beneficial to men with prostate cancer are antioxidants, they may — in theory — block the action of the radiation treatment, limiting the chance for cure. This is particularly important since recent studies have shown that cancer cells preferentially accumulate antioxidants like vitamin C and lycopene.

Although there are no human studies confirming this theory, it seems like a good idea to limit your consumption of antioxidants (vitamins E and C, lycopene and selenium) during radiation treatment. For external beam radiation, this is roughly a period of six to seven weeks. For brachytherapy, it's nine months of antioxidant abstinence (because it takes this long for palladium and iodine to lose their radioactivity within your body). Once these time periods have elapsed, you can restart nutritional supplementation.

Hormonal therapy

Many prostate cancer patients ultimately require a form of treatment known as androgen deprivation therapy (ADT). This

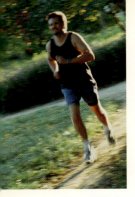

Exercise will help minimize the lean muscle loss associated with hormonal therapy.

involves blocking the production or action of testosterone and dihydrotestosterone — the two male hormones critical to prostate cell growth. These hormones are like "fuel" to prostate cancer cells. When they're removed from the circulation, the majority of prostate cancer cells will die, leading in turn to a reduction in PSA values and an improvement in the symptoms of prostate cancer such as bone pain and urinary problems.

Historically, only men with advanced bone cancer were treated with hormones. The 1990s, however, saw an increased use of hormonal therapy for men with prostate cancer. With the advent of PSA testing, men are being diagnosed with prostate cancer far earlier than before. And increasing evidence suggests that earlier treatment with ADT prolongs survival: Treating men with hormones when there's relatively less cancer is more beneficial than treating them later on when there's more cancer. Studies have also shown that, in some patients, radiation therapy can be more effective if given along with hormones.

Side-effect fighting foods

Although using hormones earlier on in treatment potentially benefits men with prostate cancer, there are some side effects associated with these drugs that relate to androgen deficiency — faster bone loss, fatigue, hot flashes, muscle-mass reduction and impotence. But nutritional and lifestyle changes may help limit some of these side effects. Here are a few suggestions:

☞ Increase your isoflavone intake to 100 mg a day. This dose will help preserve bone density and minimize hot flashes.

☞ Increase your protein intake. As outlined in Chapter 1, a complete source of low-fat protein would be best, such as soy protein.

☞ Increase the amount you exercise. Exercise, in combination with protein, will help minimize the lean muscle loss associated with ADT — and it'll also give you more energy.

☞ Eat well. A normal, balanced diet will go a long way toward helping your body cope with the physical and emotional stresses of being treated for prostate cancer.

Recipe repertoire

Now that you know which foods to eat and why, all you need is a few good recipes to get you started. So we've come up with 25 easy and tasty recipes full of healthy nutrients. In fact, many of the recipes on the following pages contain clever ways to incorporate soy products into your diet, without compromising taste — and, in many cases, even improving it. You'll also find several recipes rich in tomatoes, the main source of those all-important lycopenes.

Each recipe also has a "Prostate Cancer Nutrition Score" (one to four ⬛) that helps indicate its cancer-fighting nutritional value.

You can adapt the recipes to suit your individual tastes and preferences. For those who like to eat lighter at night, for example, many of the lunches and dinners are easily interchangeable. Or, if you don't like to cook every night, consider doubling the amounts in the recipes (especially the soups and stews) and freezing meals for later. And don't be afraid to get creative and come up with variations on your own. Before you know it, you'll be cooking up a storm — and having a great time, too.

Bon appétit!

27

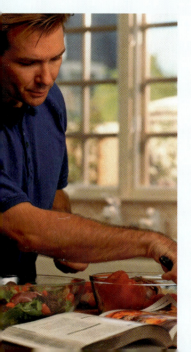

Important note:

Men who are on special diets for pre-existing health conditions, such as kidney disease or diabetes, should consult their physicians before undertaking a diet change or taking nutritional supplements.

Breakfast

Apple-Cinnamon Oatmeal
Wake up with the ultimate comfort food

¾ c. oatmeal

½ c. apples, chopped or sliced

⅛ tsp. cinnamon

1 c. plain soy milk

- Mix all ingredients in a bowl and cook, in microwave or on stove top, according to directions. Garnish with brown sugar and raisins, if desired. Can also be served cold.

Variations: Instead of apples, try oatmeal with bananas or mixed berries.

Makes 2 servings (1 cup each).

Breakfast Fruit Smoothie
A great way to get your soy

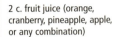

2 c. fruit juice (orange, cranberry, pineapple, apple, or any combination)

2 scoops plain or vanilla soy powder

1 c. frozen fruit (berries, peaches, mango, melon, bananas, etc.)*

- Combine all ingredients in a blender and blend until smooth.

Variation: Get creative with combinations: Try bananas with chocolate soy powder, or an all-tropical shake with pineapple juice.

Tip: While in season, freeze fresh berries and peach slices in freezer bags — it'll save you money and you'll have fresh fruit all winter long. Otherwise, frozen fruit is available in the frozen-food section of any supermarket.

Makes 2 servings.

28

Yogurt-Granola Crunch
Who cares if it's healthy? It tastes great!

¾ c. granola (preferably low-fat)

¼ c. bran buds or flakes

¼ c. nuts and raisins (optional)

¾ c. low-fat yogurt (any flavour)

¾ c. skim or soy milk

1 tbsp. honey

- Combine all ingredients in a bowl and mix well. Garnish with fresh fruit or berries, if desired. Proportions of ingredients can be adjusted according to taste.

Makes 2 servings.

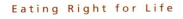

Strawberry Soy Shake
Try this sweet treat for breakfast — or dessert

- Combine all ingredients in a blender and blend until smooth.

  Makes 2 servings.

1 c. strawberry soy milk

1 c. skim milk

2 scoops vanilla or chocolate soy powder

1 c. frozen strawberries

½ c. low-fat yogurt (optional)

Tomato and Onion Scramble
Cutting back on the yolks keeps eggs on the menu

- Combine eggs, tomato, onion, tofu, oregano, salt and pepper in a bowl. Heat a heavy frying pan coated with cooking spray and add the mixture, scrambling until the eggs begin to solidify. Add cheese and cook for a few more minutes, until the desired consistency is reached.

  Makes 2 servings.

1 egg, 4 whites

½ c. chopped tomato

½ c. chopped onion

¼ c. firm-style tofu, crumbled or grated

pinch of oregano, dill or parsley (optional)

salt and pepper, to taste

low-fat butter-flavoured cooking spray

¼ c. grated low-fat mozzarella or white cheddar cheese

29

Blueberry Pancakes
Start your day the old-fashioned way

- In a large bowl, mix first three ingredients together until smooth. Add blueberries to batter and stir. Coat pan with cooking spray and heat on medium. Drop batter by large spoonfuls onto pan. Cook until edges are dry, then flip. Cook until golden.

  Makes 2 servings.

1 c. pancake mix, preferably buckwheat or other grain (not refined flour)

1 ½ - 2 c. plain soy milk or skim milk

1 egg (with or without yolk)

¾ c. blueberries

low-fat butter-flavoured cooking spray

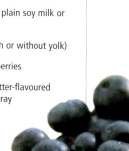

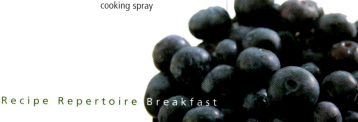

Lunch

Leek and Green Bean Soup
A hearty favourite that's good for you, too

1 lb. (450 g) green beans

4 c. vegetable or chicken stock

2 leeks, white and light-green parts only

3 tsp. olive oil

1 ½ tbsp. flour

½ c. soy or skim milk

salt and pepper, to taste

• Cut beans into 1-inch pieces. Place in a large saucepan and add vegetable stock. Bring to a boil, reduce heat and simmer. Meanwhile, dice leeks in half lengthwise, wash thoroughly and cut into 1-inch pieces. Heat oil in a large frying pan and sauté leeks until soft, a few minutes. Add flour to leeks, stirring constantly. Cook for a minute or two.

• Add the leek mixture to the soup with beans and bring to a boil, whisking. Reduce heat and simmer 30 minutes. Purée the soup in a blender or food processor. Return to the saucepan. Stir in milk, salt and pepper. Heat again thoroughly before serving.

Serves 4.

30

No-Fuss Cabbage Rolls
Stuff 'em with beef, chicken or, better yet, tofu

(if made with tofu)

4 c. shredded cabbage

1 lb. (450 g) crumbled firm-style tofu, extra-lean ground beef or chicken

1 large onion, finely chopped

¾ tsp. garlic powder

½ tsp. salt

⅔ c. uncooked long-grain rice

3 ½ c. tomato juice

⅓ c. chili sauce or ketchup

• In a large 10-cup (2.5-L) casserole, layer a third of the cabbage, half of each of the tofu or meat, onion, garlic powder, salt and rice. Pour 1 cup of the tomato juice over layers. Add a second layer of the six ingredients and then another cup of tomato juice. Top with remaining cabbage. Stir chili sauce into remaining tomato juice; pour over casserole.

• Bake, covered, in 325°F (165°C) oven for 1 1/2 to 2 hours.

Makes 8 servings.

Super Stuffed Tomatoes
Perfect for lunch, or as a side dish with supper

- Cut off tops of tomatoes. Using a teaspoon, scrape out the flesh of each tomato and reserve. Arrange tomatoes in an oven-proof dish and set aside.

- Boil pasta according to instructions. In a large saucepan coated with vegetable spray, sauté vegetables with garlic until tender. Add half of the tomato centres and cook until liquid reduces. Add breadcrumbs, pasta, salt and pepper.

- Preheat oven to 400°F (205°C). Stuff each tomato with the mixture, placing any extras on the bottom of the dish, and bake for about 20 minutes or until heated through.

Serves four.

4 large beefsteak tomatoes

⅔ c. miniature pasta (any shape)

low-fat non-stick vegetable spray

1 celery stalk, chopped

2 small cloves garlic

½ c. sliced mushrooms

2 shallots, chopped

⅓ c. breadcrumbs

salt and pepper, to taste

31

Goat Cheese Pita Wraps
A more daring version of the standard grilled-cheese sandwich

- Open pita entirely, separate sides and spread cheese evenly over each half. Cover with lettuce, onion and tomato. Roll each side tightly into a wrap and secure with a toothpick. Can also be served warm.

Serves two.

1 large whole-wheat pita

low-fat goat cheese (spread or slices)

lettuce

1 small red onion, thinly sliced

1 tomato, thinly sliced

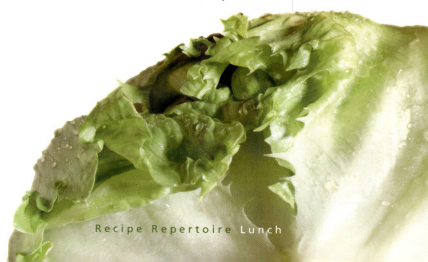

Lunch

Sweet Potato Stew
A meal in a bowl, packed with nutrients, soy and lycopenes

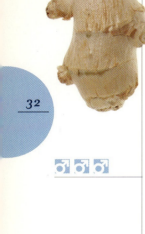

2 c. chopped onion

1/2 tsp. cayenne or chili pepper

1-2 tsp. pressed garlic

1 tbsp. flaxseed or vegetable oil

2 c. chopped cabbage

3 c. cubed sweet potatoes

3 c. tomato juice

1 c. apple juice

1 tsp. salt

1 tsp. ginger (powdered or fresh grated)

2 tomatoes, chopped

1 c. cubed tofu, firm style

In a large frying pan, brown onions, chili pepper and garlic in oil. Add cabbage and sweet potatoes and sauté, covered, for a few minutes. Mix in apple and tomato juices, salt, ginger, tomatoes and tofu. Cover and simmer for 15 to 30 minutes, until potatoes are tender. Serve with whole-wheat rolls.

Variation: Add a cup of green vegetables, like green beans, broccoli, okra or brussels sprouts.

Makes 4-6 servings.

32

Wheat Germ Burgers
They taste better than they sound — guaranteed!

1 egg, 2 whites

1/2 c. toasted wheat germ*

1/2 c. bread crumbs

1/2 c. sliced shallots

1/2 c. crumbled firm-style tofu

2 tbsp. parsley

1/2 tsp. paprika

1/2 tsp. oregano

1/4 c. chopped mushrooms

* available in most grocery and health food stores.

In a large bowl, mix all ingredients until well combined. Form into 4 patties and broil in the oven or grill on the barbecue until cooked through. Top burgers with a slice of low-fat cheese, sweet onion, lettuce and serve on whole-wheat buns.

Makes 4 burgers.

Roasted Veggie Baguette
A sandwich that'll inspire you to grow your own garden

- Slice all vegetables thinly. Spray cookie sheet lined with tin foil. Arrange vegetables and garlic on sheet and roast until soft, about 30 minutes, turning vegetables occasionally to combine flavours.

- Cut baguette in half and scoop out some of the dough, then fill pockets with vegetables. Serve warm or cold. During the summer, vegetables can be grilled on the barbecue for added flavour.

Makes two servings.

½ red pepper

½ eggplant

1 c. mushrooms

1 small zucchini

1 sweet onion

3 cloves garlic

1 whole-wheat baguette

low-fat non-stick vegetable spray

33

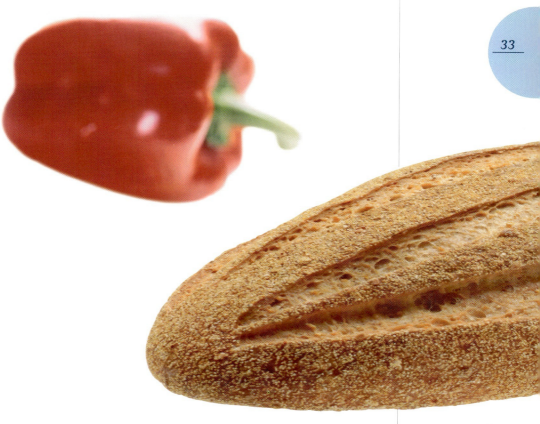

Dinner

Spinach and Mushroom Lasagna
Leave out the meat for a healthier version of this Italian favourite

2 cloves garlic, crushed

1 large onion, chopped

1 lb. (450 g) mushrooms, sliced

1 ½ lb. (675 g) frozen spinach, thawed and drained (fresh spinach can be substituted)

approx. 3 c. thick tomato sauce

½ lb. (225 g) fresh or packaged whole-wheat lasagna noodles, cooked

1 ½ c. grated low-fat mozzarella cheese

• In a large skillet, sauté the garlic, onion and mushrooms until tender. Add spinach and cook for about 5 minutes. To assemble the lasagna, spread 1/2 c. of tomato sauce on the bottom of a 9-inch square baking dish and cover with 1/3 of noodles. Add half the spinach mixture, 3/4 c. tomato sauce, and 1/2 c. of cheese. Cover with another layer of noodles and repeat the process. Top with a final layer of noodles, 3/4 c. tomato sauce and cheese. Cover with aluminum foil and bake for 30 minutes at 375°F (190°C). Remove foil and cook an additional 15 minutes.

Variation: Add 1 c. crumbled firm-style tofu to the spinach mixture.

Makes 4 servings.

Crispy Salmon Steaks
You don't have to be a fish fan to love these fillets

2 6-oz. salmon steaks

2 egg whites

1 tbsp. lemon juice

½ c. cornflake crumbs

½ c. grated Parmesan cheese

salt and pepper, to taste

2 tsp. dried dill

2 tsp. dried parsley

low-fat butter-flavoured cooking spray

• Mix egg and lemon juice together on a plate. Dip both sides of salmon steaks into egg mixture, then firmly press steaks into mixture of crumbs, cheese, salt, pepper, dill and parsley, making sure they're well coated. Refrigerate at least 1 hour. Place steaks on aluminum foil coated with cooking spray and broil for 5 minutes on each side. Serves 2.

34

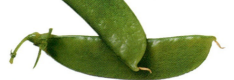

Raspberry Vinegar Chicken

Impress your guests with this elegant, high-protein dish

- Cut chicken into 2-inch chunks. Pat dry and dust with flour. Heat oil in large non-stick saucepan. Cook chicken for about 5 minutes, turning it over as necessary. Sprinkle with salt, pepper and Italian seasoning. Remove chicken and set aside (keep warm).

- Steam snow peas or other vegetables.

- Sauté shallots for a minute in the same pan and add the raspberry vinegar and wine. Cook on high heat, scraping pan until sauce has reduced slightly. Return chicken to pan, turning to absorb the sauce. Add snow peas and tomatoes, and heat thoroughly. Serve over rice.

Serves 4.

1 lb. (450 g) skinless, boneless chicken breasts

¼ c. all-purpose flour

1 tbsp. flaxseed or vegetable oil

¼ c. chopped shallots

½ tsp. Italian seasoning of any kind

¼ c. dry white wine or chicken stock

¼ c. raspberry vinegar

1 c. or more snow peas (or other vegetables)

2 tomatoes cut into eighths, or 10 cherry tomatoes

salt and pepper, to taste

35

Classic Tofu Stir-Fry

An Asian-inspired one-dish meal that's sure to satisfy

- Over medium-high heat, lightly coat a wok or large frying pan with cooking spray. Add tofu, garlic and ginger and cook, stirring, until tofu is slightly browned. Add mushrooms and onions and cook, stirring, until lightly browned.

- Add pepper, carrots, bok choy and sauce (mix soy sauce, teriyaki sauce, vinegar, honey, stock and water). Stir over medium to high heat until sauce bubbles and thickens and carrots are cooked through. Serve over brown rice.

Makes 2 generous servings.

1 package firm-style tofu, cut into cubes

2 cloves garlic, crushed

1 tsp. ginger, finely minced

4-6 shiitake mushrooms, sliced

1 medium onion, chopped

1 green or red pepper, chopped

2 carrots, diced

1 c. bok choy, chopped

non-stick cooking spray

3 tbsp. lite soy sauce

⅛ c. teriyaki sauce

1 tbsp. rice vinegar

1 tbsp. honey

⅓ c. vegetable stock

¼ c. water

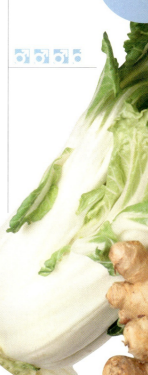

Dinner

Foil-Baked Fish Parmigiana
Short on time? This prostate-friendly entrée is ready in minutes

4 6-oz. fish fillets, any kind

7 ½-oz. can of tomato sauce

salt and ground black pepper, to taste

½ c. chopped onion

½ c. sliced mushrooms

½ c. grated low-fat Parmesan cheese

low-fat butter-flavoured cooking spray

- Place each serving of fish in the centre of a large sheet of aluminum foil sprayed with non-stick cooking spray; cup foil around fish. Sprinkle each serving with salt and pepper.

- Spread tomato sauce, onion and mushrooms over each serving and sprinkle with cheese.

- Pull foil edges together; seal well, leaving small air space inside.

- Preheat oven to 400°F (205°C) and bake for 20 minutes or until fish flakes easily when tested with a fork.

Makes 4 servings.

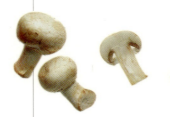

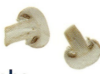

Turkey and Tofu Kabobs
Fire up the barbecue for these smart skewers

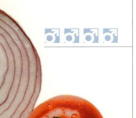

1 large boneless turkey breast, cubed

½ package firm-style tofu, cut into large cubes

8 cherry tomatoes

8 pearl onions

1 bottle low-fat Italian salad dressing

- In a shallow dish, marinate all ingredients in salad dressing for at least two hours or overnight in the refrigerator. Arrange ingredients on 4 to 6 skewers and place in broiling pan.

- Barbecue or broil, uncovered, basting with remaining marinade and turning skewers once or twice, until done.

Serves 2.

36

Sweet and Spicy Tomato Sauce with Tofu
A tasty new twist on an old classic

In a large saucepan over medium heat in hot oil, add tofu and brown garlic and onion. Stir in chili sauce, tomato juice, tomato paste and remaining ingredients. Reduce heat to low, partially cover and simmer sauce 35 to 45 minutes, stirring occasionally. Remove bay leaf before serving. Serve over whole-wheat pasta.

Variations: Lean ground beef or chicken can be substituted for tofu — just remember to drain the fat after browning the meat. Another option is to add Nutballs (recipe page 40) to the sauce before serving.

Makes 4 servings.

2 tbsp. flaxseed or vegetable oil

1 lb. (450 g) pre-packaged ground tofu or crumbled firm-style tofu

2 cloves garlic, minced

1 medium onion, chopped

1 bottle (285 mL) chili sauce

2 c. tomato juice

2 tbsp. tomato paste

1 tsp. basil

1 tsp. oregano

1 tsp. salt

1 tsp. marjoram (optional)

1 bay leaf

37

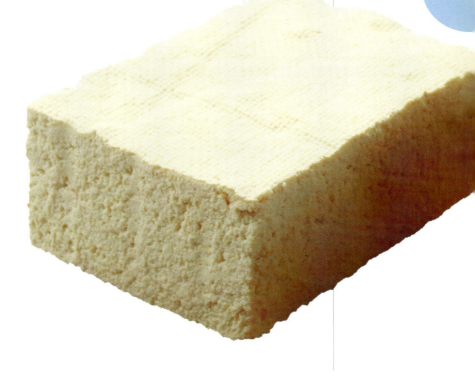

Dessert

Chocolate Mousse
Finally! A guilt-free way to indulge your sweet tooth

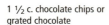

1 ½ c. chocolate chips or grated chocolate

2 tsp. butter or oil

¼ c. water

1 tbsp. unflavoured gelatin

½ c. cold water

1 c. soft tofu

¼ c. liqueur (amaretto, crème de menthe, etc.)

1 tsp. vanilla extract

dash of salt

• Combine chocolate, butter and 1/4 c. water in a heavy-bottomed saucepan, stirring constantly over medium heat until the mixture is melted and smooth. Lower heat. In a small bowl, mix gelatin with 1/2 c. cold water, then add to chocolate mixture in pan. Stir constantly until gelatin disappears completely. Remove from heat. In a blender or food processor, combine tofu, liqueur, vanilla and salt. Add to chocolate mixture and blend until smooth. Pour into 4 to 6 cups and refrigerate several hours, until set.

38

Clafouti
Fruit and custard create a heavenly combination

1 lb. (450 g) fruit (cherries, plums, peaches or berries)

½ c. sifted flour

⅔ c. sugar (or slightly less)

pinch of salt

2 eggs, 2 whites

1 ½ c. soy or 1% milk

3 tbsp. butter, melted and cooled

• Wash and dry fruit, slice if required, or drain if preserved or frozen. In a large bowl, combine flour, 1/2 c. (or less) sugar and the salt. Add slightly beaten eggs, blending thoroughly with whisk. Add milk and melted butter, stirring until smooth (do not heat).

• Butter a 9-inch square baking pan. Sprinkle 1 tbsp. of sugar. Spread fruit on bottom then pour in batter.

• Preheat oven to 400°F (205°C). Bake for 30 minutes. Sprinkle top with remaining sugar. Continue baking for another 15 minutes or until custard is firm.

Serves 4 to 6.

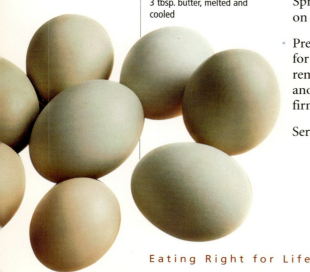

Apple-Blueberry Crumble
Dessert the way grandma used to make it

- Spread sliced apples, blueberries and raisins in an oven-proof casserole coated with cooking spray. Mix oatmeal, brown sugar and nuts in a small bowl and spread the mixture over the top of the fruit. Preheat oven to 350°F (175°C) and bake for approximately 30 minutes, or until bubbly and the nuts are golden and the apples cooked. Serve with vanilla ice cream or frozen-tofu dessert.

Serves 4.

4-5 apples, peeled and sliced

1 1/2 c. blueberries

1/4 c. raisins

1/2 c. oatmeal

1/4 c. brown sugar

1/4 c. slivered almonds or brazil nuts

low-fat butter-flavoured cooking spray

39

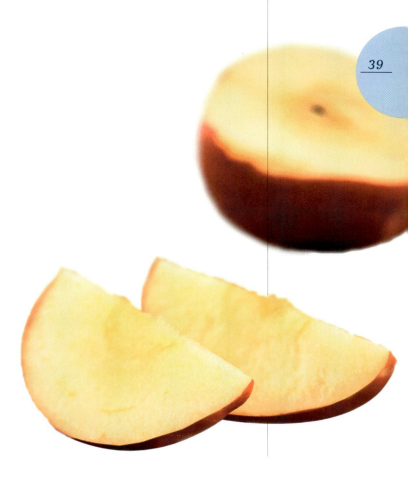

Appetizers and Snacks

Nutballs
A versatile — and delicious — substitute for meatballs

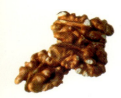

1 c. whole-wheat bread or cracker crumbs

¾ c. grated low-fat cheddar cheese

¾ c. finely chopped pecans

1 egg, 2 whites beaten

1 small onion, minced

1 clove garlic, minced

1 tbsp. chopped fresh parsley

1 tsp. soy sauce

½ tsp. ground sage

½ tsp. pepper

non-stick cooking spray

• Preheat oven to 350°F (175°C). In a large bowl, combine all of the ingredients and stir well. Form the mixture into about 36 balls the size of walnuts.

• Place the balls on a baking sheet coated with cooking spray. Bake until lightly browned, about 15 minutes, turning about halfway through. If preferred, balls may be browned in a skillet.

• Nutballs can be served as a side dish or as an appetizer with tomato sauce or peanut sauce for dipping, or substituted for meatballs along with spaghetti.

Serves about 4.

40

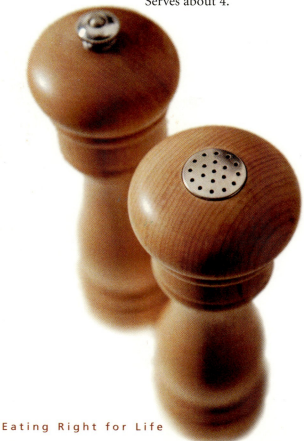